About
You
... and other
important people

About
You
... and other
important people

Glen C. Griffin, M.D., and Mary Ella Griffin, R.N.

Illustrated by Heidi Darley

Deseret Book Company
Salt Lake City, Utah
1980

Library of Congress Cataloging in Publication Data

Griffin, Glen C
    About you . . . and other important people.

    SUMMARY: Basic information about reproduction,
growth of a baby, and birth, emphasizing the
importance of moral sexual behavior from a Mormon
point of view.
    1. Sex instruction for children. [1. Sex
instruction for children. 2. Sexual ethics]
I. Griffin, Mary Ella, 1936-   joint author.
II. Title.
HQ53.G67   301.41'07   79-17256
ISBN 0-87747-752-3

Especially for Jill and Greg . . .
and all their friends, everywhere

Contents

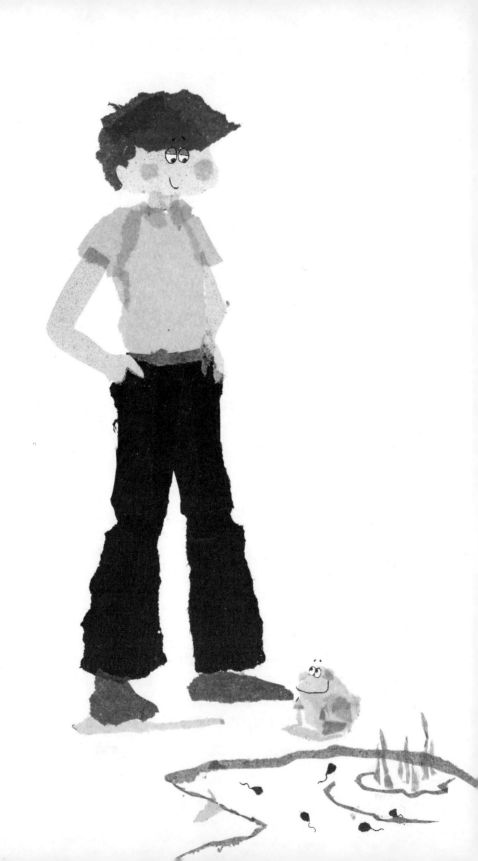

About You

This book is about an interesting and important person . . . YOU!

You already know a lot about a lot of things, such as how to fix a sandwich, what to do in case of a fire, and how to spend money quickly. You know about laws and rules. You probably know quite a bit about math and spelling. You know about people, places, and things. You know that some people are always loyal friends, while others are sometimes hard to understand.

You know that you have a Heavenly Father. You know that your spirit-self is a child of heavenly parents. And you also know that you were born of earthly parents because your spirit needed an earthly body.

Yet many people in the world don't have

1

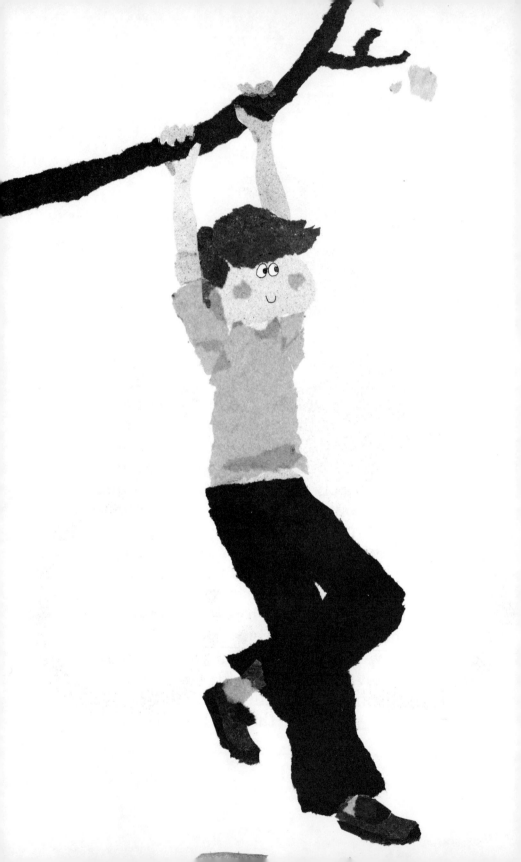

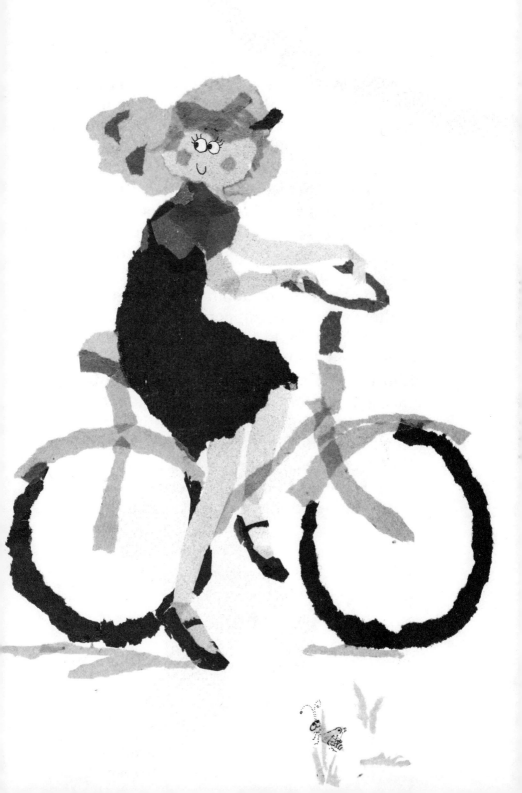

any idea what life is really about. This is one reason some people make such big mistakes about important things. And when people don't know why we are here on earth, or about forever families, they may have wrong answers about marriage, and babies, and other things.

When you have questions about your birth, your life, or your body, ask your mom or dad. They can be very comforting when things seem mixed-up and confusing.

This book is not about fish or dogs, bees or elephants, birds or hippopotamuses. This book is about you. It is about how your earth life began, and how the earth lives of your own children will begin. This book is about sperm and eggs and how they get together. Knowing how you were born is more important than knowing about fish or bees or elephants or any other creatures. It is important to know what is going on in your body, and why. So this book is about you—and other important people.

Your
Body
Is a
Wonderful
Machine

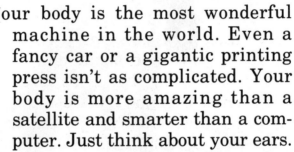our body is the most wonderful machine in the world. Even a fancy car or a gigantic printing press isn't as complicated. Your body is more amazing than a satellite and smarter than a computer. Just think about your ears. Sound waves hit your eardrums. Then tiny bones vibrate, sending the sound on its way to the inner ear and then to the brain. And what about your feet? Have you ever thought about the tendons, muscles, bones, nerves, ligaments, and blood vessels that make up a foot?

Your body is made up of millions and millions of cells. Some are large. Some are small. Some are blood cells. Some are muscle cells. Some are bone cells. Some make insulin. Other cells are ova and others are sperm. Why do

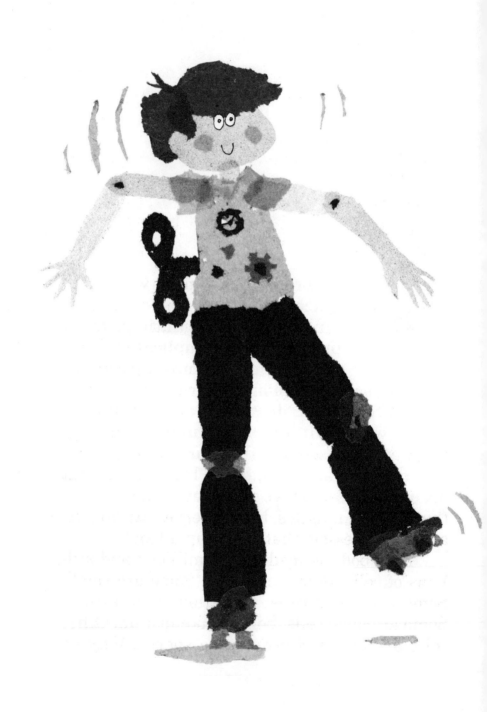

some cells become specialists to do one thing, and others to do something else? Why do cells divide into more cells the way they do? How do they know when to stop and when to start? How do they know when and how to do all the things they do?

No one knows all the answers. But the human body is amazing. What a magnificent home it is for your spirit!

No one can make a computer like your brain. No one can make a heart that is anything like your heart, even though scientists have developed artificial hearts that can act as substitutes for a little while. No one can make a machine do the thousands of things your fingers and hands can do, and the finest cameras cannot compare with your eyes.

Have you ever thought about your spleen or pancreas? Do you know what they do to keep your body going as it should? There are probably many other body parts that you've never heard of or thought about. Yet each part keeps doing its job, day after day.

The more we study the body, the more amazing we find it to be. A machine runs on a certain kind of fuel, but the body's energy system can run on several different fuels. Although the body works best with a variety of nourishing foods, it will run at least for a while on almost anything you feed it—spinach, potatoes, milk, rice or hamburgers and ice cream.

Some things are very harmful to this complicated machine of ours, such as tobacco, alcohol, and many other drugs. Putting such things in one's body makes as little sense as putting salt or dirt in the gas tank of an automobile.

If you were to begin studying about your body right now and were to continue this project all your life, you would never learn everything there is to know about it. You may not want to spend a lifetime learning about your body, but almost everyone wants to learn something about how it works and the amazing things it can do.

Especially interesting are the questions about birth, and how a cell from a father and a cell from a mother join to grow into a baby. Compared with all the things your body can do, this is one of the most amazing. A sperm from a father meets an ovum (egg) from a mother. Let's explore these questions and others, starting with some interesting things about boys, and then we'll look at the special qualities of girls.

About
Boys

Boys come equipped with hair, eyes, lots of bones, millions of brain cells, muscles, a heart, and some special organs that make it possible for them to someday become fathers. Of course, boys are very different from girls. Each boy is also very different from every other boy. One boy may be a really good ball player. Another may be more interested in electronics and computers. Some boys can run faster, some can jump farther, and some are better in math. One thing for sure is that every boy can be *the best* in something.

Sometimes a boy doesn't know this. Often he doesn't even think about himself as being the best in anything. But almost for sure he is. He may be the best friend. He may be the kind-

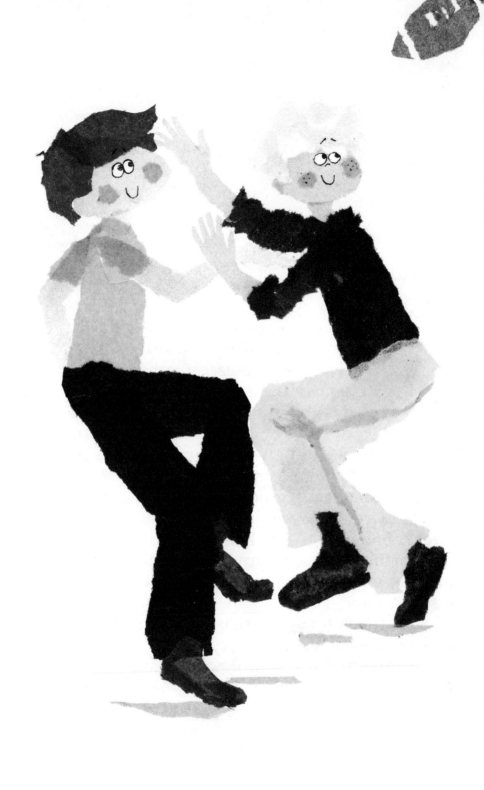

est boy in the neighborhood. He may be willing to listen when someone has a problem. He may become a good musician, inventor, or writer. He may become a great missionary or a leader in the Church.

Have you ever thought about what a boy might do in his lifetime? He might someday become a military captain or even a general. He might become a governor, a senator, or maybe even president. But more important than all of these, he will very likely become a father. He can also become an eternal father. As you think about a particular boy, or as you think about yourself, these thoughts may be startling, but they are true. A boy may not reach this potential, but it is possible. And that is what life is all about.

There are some tough tests. There are some difficult requirements. But along with them there are lots of fun things for a boy to do as he grows up, such as eating, exploring, building, competing, thinking, learning, discovering, and even working. There are some serious times, some spiritual moments, some upsets and disasters. But along the way the bumps and bruises somehow make him stronger and perhaps even wiser. The boy you know best probably has failed a few times already, but he has been able to get up and get going again.

One of the most important things about a boy is his ability to become a father. If he controls this power and uses it properly, he will have passed one of the most important tests in life.

How does this power to become a father work? As a boy grows into a man many changes occur. He grows taller in spurts. For a while no growth seems to happen at all. Then about the time he wears a new pair of pants a few times it becomes obvious that they are already too small. This may happen quite a few times during a period of fast growth. His voice may squeak and crack as it changes into the deeper sound of a man. During this time there may be some embarrassing moments when he talks or sings. One moment his voice is that of a man, and the next that of a boy, and then in mid-sentence it changes again.

Soon whiskers begin to grow, and hair begins to grow between his legs. Soon his body produces tiny sperm cells, which under a microscope look like tiny tadpoles. Each of these little cells has a constantly wiggling tail. Sperm are produced in two organs called testicles, each of which is about the size of a pecan. They are found between the upper legs in a skin

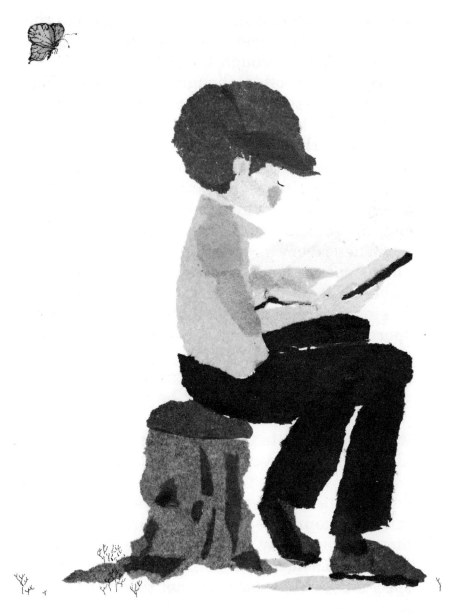

sac called the scrotum. As the boy matures the testicles produce sperm. Eventually the sperm leave the body through the penis.

Sperm are often thought of as seeds. But they are somewhat different from seeds. Seeds need only be planted in soil, where, if nourished, they will grow into whatever they are supposed to become, such as carrots, melons, tomatoes, or beans. But a sperm must join a female's ovum, which is sometimes called an egg, in order to grow into a person.

When a boy reaches maturity and is producing sperm, it is possible for him to become a father. But he is not yet ready to be a father. There is more to being a father than providing sperm. A father needs to be responsible. He must be married. He must obey the Lord's sacred commandments. The scriptures say that a male and female may only be joined together when they are married to each other. A boy will want to be sure that he never lets anyone tempt him to break this commandment.

Each boy has the potential to become a father. The special powers are there—but they must be controlled and used properly. This means that a boy must not allow himself or anyone else to touch or play with his body's special parts. He also must not touch or tamper

14

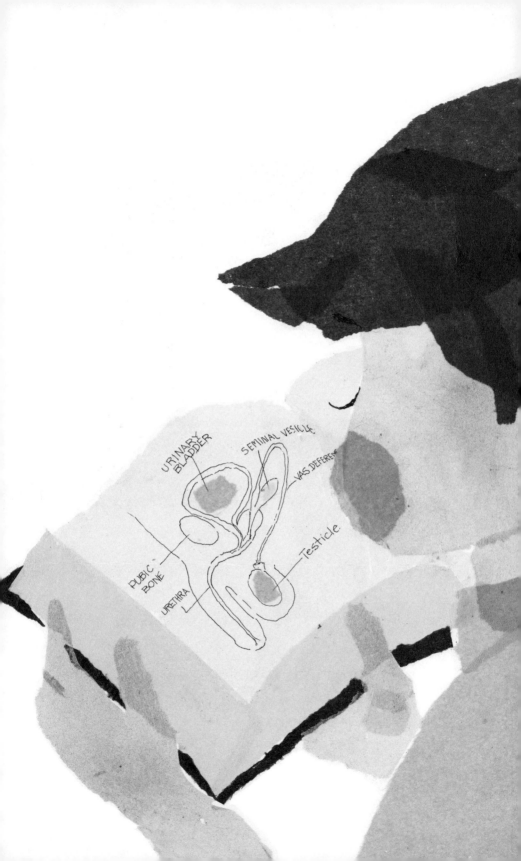

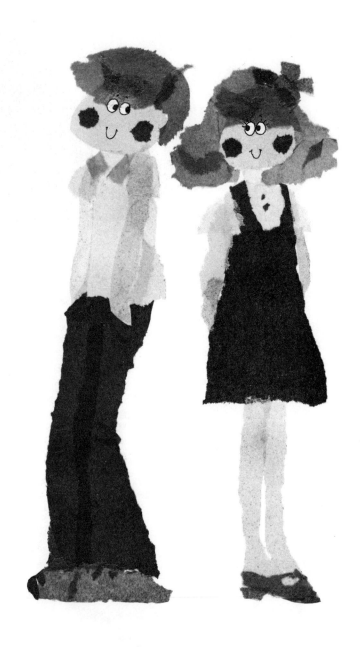

with anyone else's sacred body parts.

In many ways boys are difficult to describe. You will be learning more about boys all your life, little by little, about how they think, how they act, what they like and don't like, and many other things. Always keep in mind, though, the potential of a boy. As each day comes and goes, a boy is always making choices. He really can choose to be and to do what he wants.

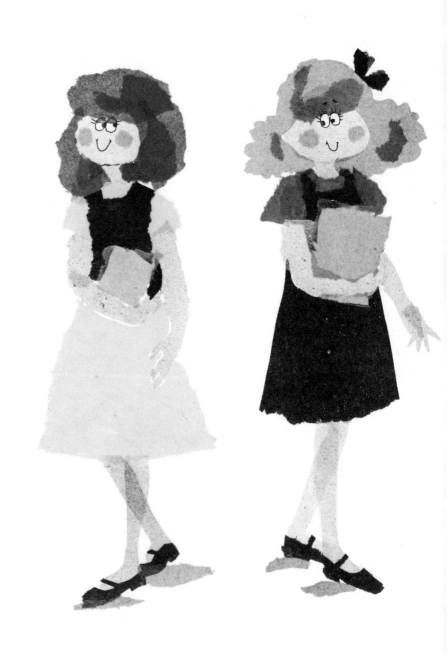

About Girls

Pony tails, perfume, ribbons, giggles, records, and hairbrushes and parties may all come to mind when one thinks about girls. But a girl is much more than a giggling creature with some records in one hand and a hairbrush in the other. Every girl is a precious child of God. Every girl is an individual. Every girl has some special qualities that no one else has.

Just as a boy needs to recognize his own talents, so also does a girl. Every girl can be the best in a special way. Even a girl with many problems can have the sweetest smile, the most pleasant disposition, and many other positive qualities. And looking ahead, a girl can someday become a wife and mother, and even an eternal mother, the companion to an eternal father.

Girls are interesting creations. Most of them have two ears, ten toes, a pancreas, lots of bones and blood vessels, and nerves and skin. In some ways a girl's body is very much like a boy's. But in many other ways her body is also very different. Amazing as it may seem, even little girls in bluejeans can become lovely, grown-up young women.

Sometime when a girl is between the ages of nine and fourteen, a little bump appears on one or both sides of her chest. Each bump may be somewhat tender and bothersome. The girl may think something is wrong, and even a knowing mother may be surprised and alarmed. These little bumps may be the first sign that other changes are coming. A little body hair begins to appear, and the firm little bumps on each side of her chest slowly change to soft curves. As these and other important changes are taking place, both inside and out, a girl may often find that tears appear in her eyes and run down her cheeks almost without warning. She worries about changes, about growing up, and about changes in her feelings and her body that she doesn't understand. Some of her tears may be tears of joy, but others may be

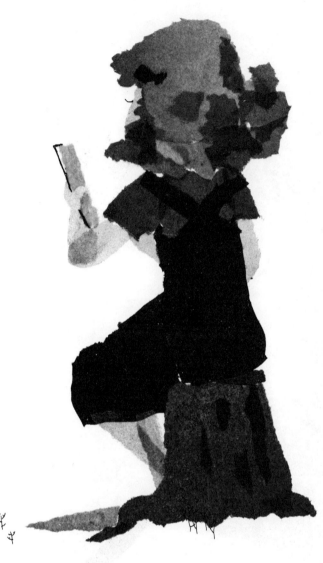

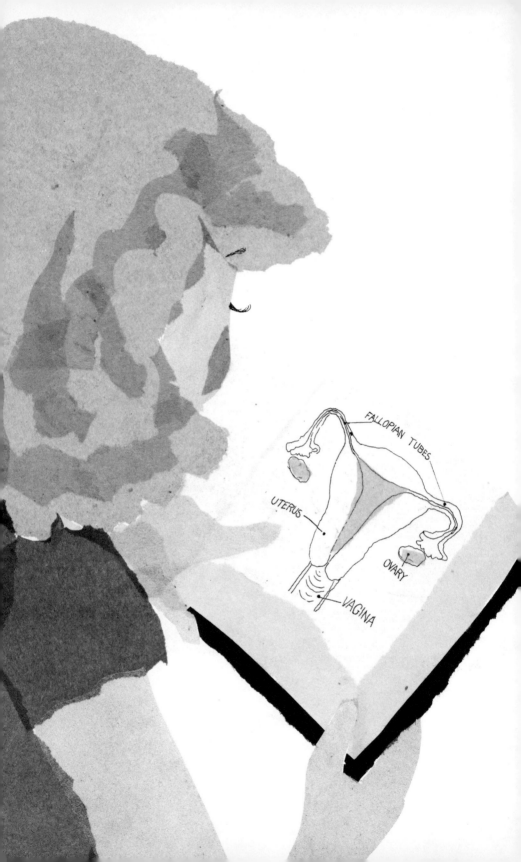

FALLOPIAN TUBES

UTERUS

OVARY

VAGINA

tears of frustration and bewilderment.

As brothers and friends wonder what is happening, history repeats itself as a girl changes into a woman. One day at twelve, eleven, or maybe not until fifteen, some special parts inside her body will have developed enough so that another exciting event occurs. Menstruation begins. Some spots of blood and tissue in the uterus are no longer needed, and are discharged from the body. Every month or so, for many years, this will happen for three to five days at a time. Why?

Approximately every twenty-eight days an ovum, or egg, is released from one of a female's ovaries. Since birth, a lifetime supply of these eggs has been stored in the ovaries, which are well protected inside the girl's body, one on each side. Each ovary is connected to the uterus by a fallopian tube. Each month a tiny ovum or egg is released from the ovary. The ovum makes its way down the fallopian tube into the uterus, where a baby can grow. The uterus becomes prepared every month to accept an egg that has joined with a sperm. But when an egg is not joined with a sperm, the egg is discarded along with the lining cells of the uterus. These cells, along with some blood, leave the uterus and flow out of the girl's body through the cer-

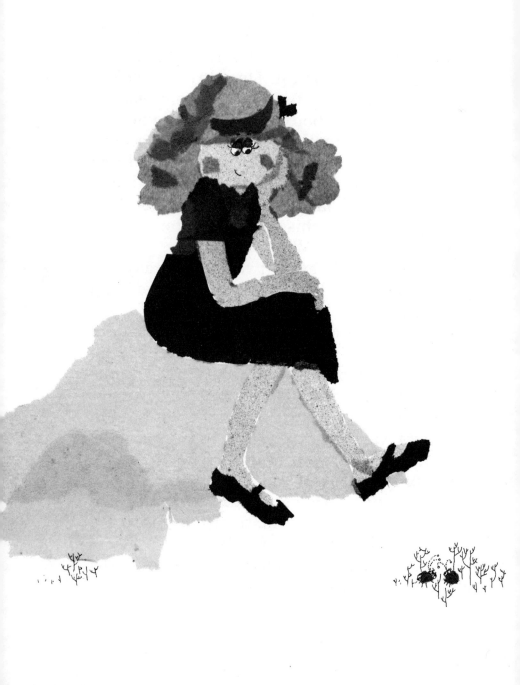

vix and vagina. This is called a menstrual period. While this bleeding is occurring, a pad is worn to take care of the discharge.

What a wonderful experience it is for a girl to know that her body is being prepared for motherhood, even though she is not really ready to become a mother for several more years. During these years she can be preparing herself spiritually, intellectually, and physically for the day when this miracle will take place.

This preparation time can be a choice time in a girl's life, as she learns how to become a better person and how to prepare for the future. Earth life and eternal life are adventures. How each girl's particular adventure turns out is up to her. Day by day, as she creates her own life story, she can enjoy a whole new world in which she learns to understand other people and to become less selfish. She will be faced with some puzzling problems and decisions. There will be days full of joy and excitement and, of course, other times that don't seem interesting or happy at all. These ups and downs can be handled more easily if one knows some of the really important things in life and eternity.

As a girl looks ahead she must decide what the really important things are and how she

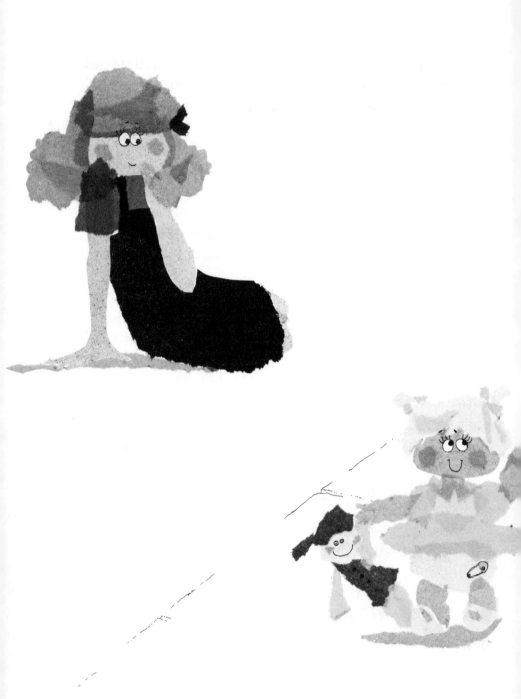

will prepare herself to handle them. Most girls look ahead to many fun and interesting things to do, including falling in love and marrying someone very special, and having a family. Getting married is exciting. So is the special experience of becoming a mother. Loving, teaching, and bringing up children are as challenging as any career.

But while being a mother is exciting, it is also difficult and requires much preparation. That is why a girl must resist any temptation to have experiences that should be reserved for marriage. She must not allow herself or anyone else to touch special parts of her body. She also must not touch or tamper with anyone else's special body parts. Allowing anyone to play with or experiment with one's special body parts can lead to serious problems. Such actions are not appropriate for a future eternal mother.

These choice years of growing up should be fun years. As a girl grows up she usually does a lot of thinking—about things that will happen today and tomorrow, but also about what kind of person she will become, and the kind of person she wants to live with forever. Many movies or television shows would have her believe that such decisions can be made quickly—but such shows are not about people who are looking forward to a forever marriage. Unlike many of the stories in movies or TV, everyday living in marriage can be wonderful. And a girl's adventure can continue forever. She and her husband can have an eternal family—he as an eternal father and she as an eternal mother.

Of course, in order to obtain such very special opportunities, a girl must qualify. How? The requirements are spelled out clearly in the scriptures.

A girl who is going to become an eternal mother is a special person. Only in marriage will she share her body with someone else, remaining clean and pure for her husband. Then, at the proper time, under the proper circumstances, she can share herself with him.

Girls are wonderful. No one could possibly know or explain all about them. They can be soft and lovely. They can be gentle and kind. They must be treated with respect by themselves and others. Every girl is precious in many, many ways, and has great and wonderful adventures ahead.

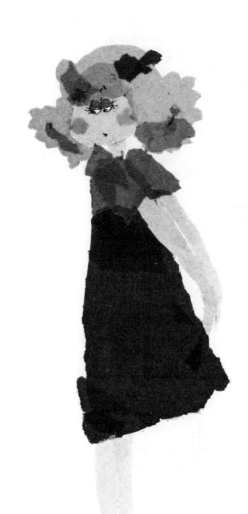

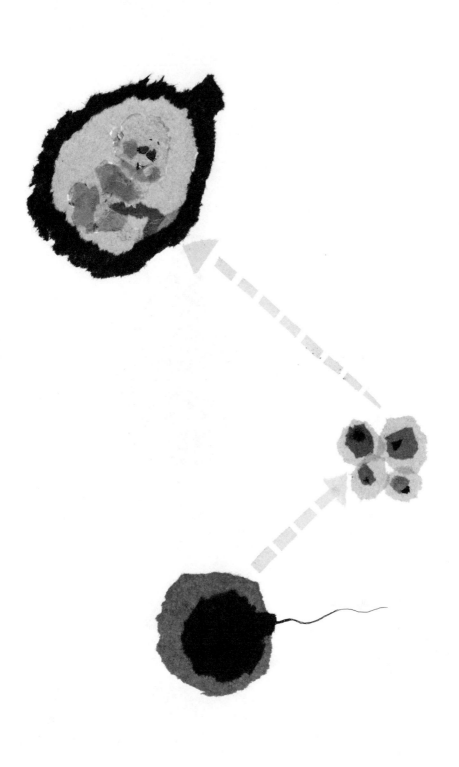

A Sperm and an Ovum Get Together

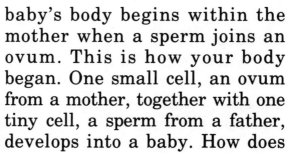 baby's body begins within the mother when a sperm joins an ovum. This is how your body began. One small cell, an ovum from a mother, together with one tiny cell, a sperm from a father, develops into a baby. How does this happen?

The scriptures tell us, "Therefore shall a man leave his father and his mother, and shall cleave unto his wife: and they shall be one flesh." (Genesis 2:24.) What does this mean? How does the sperm get from the father into the mother? For this to happen, two people must be so close together that their bodies are, as the scripture says, "one flesh." A part of the father is within a part of the mother. This is a very special time.

Joining bodies is so sacred that only a husband and his wife should ever be together in this way. This is called mating. It is also called intercourse. The sperm travel through the penis of the father into the vagina of the mother. This is a very sacred and private experience. A man's and woman's body parts must be joined together only in marriage. A boy and girl or man and woman must never be together in this way until they are married to each other. There must be no tampering with these special body parts outside of marriage.

When sperm do enter the vagina, millions of them swim rapidly in all directions. Some of the sperm find their way up through the cervix and into the uterus. Then some of them continue to find their way into the fallopian tubes. If an egg or ovum is present, sperm are attracted to it. When a sperm joins an egg, the egg becomes fertilized and is called a zygote. This is how a baby's body begins.

Often the egg is not joined by a sperm, and thus it remains unfertilized. However, when the egg is fertilized, the zygote journeys down the fallopian tube and finds a warm, comfortable home in the uterus, in a specially prepared lining called the endometrium.

Here the zygote divides into two cells and

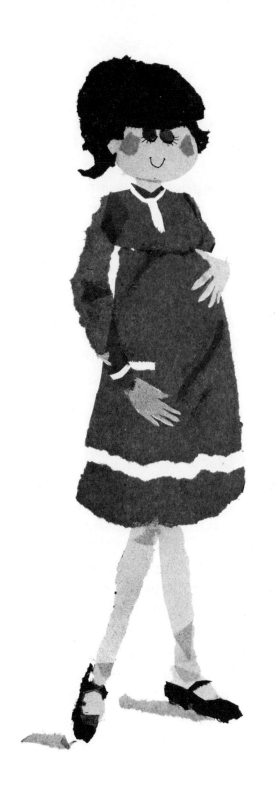

they divide into four, and the four cells divide
into eight, and so on until millions-upon-
millions of cells have developed into the various
parts and complicated organs of a minute little
baby. Growth and further development continue for about nine months, with the baby living in a sac of protective fluid, usually in an
upside-down position within the uterus.

You may wonder why the baby doesn't
drown, being completely covered with fluid.
This cannot happen because the baby doesn't
start to breathe through his nose and mouth
until he is born and takes his first breath, ex-
panding his lungs for the first time.

The developing baby receives all his
nourishment from the mother through a special
system of blood vessels in the placenta, which
transfers food and oxygen from the mother to
the baby. These vessels go through the umbilical cord, which connects the baby at the navel
to the mother.

Imagine the amazing things that happen
during these months in the uterus. The baby's
arms and legs form, and so do the heart and
lungs. Eyes develop that are so intricate that no
one can make anything like them. Some cells
develop into a brain, and others into bones to be
a framework for the body. Still others form

muscle, blood, ears, and on and on. All this is really unbelievable—yet it all really happens. Then after nine months, or sometimes a little less, a baby is ready to be born. A body has been prepared. Now it is time for the adventure of earth life to begin. But how is a baby born?

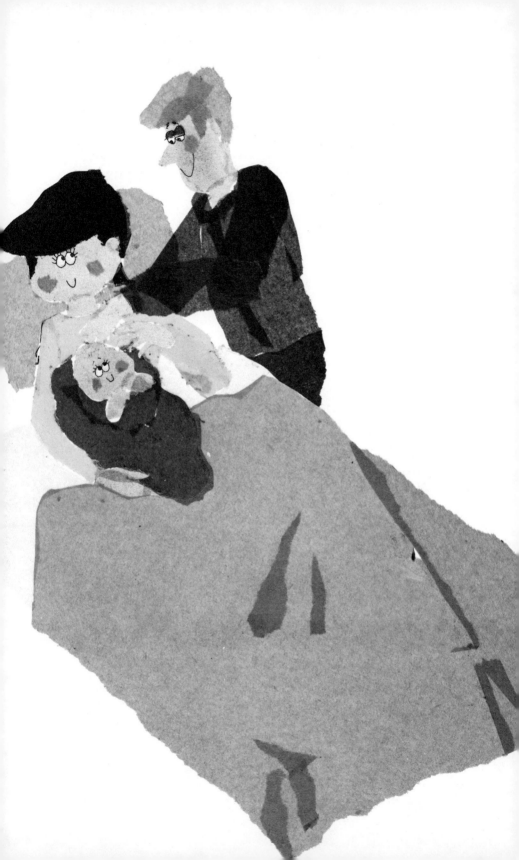

A
Baby
Is
Born

In the nine months or so since the sperm met the ovum, there has been a big change. Now the baby weighs about seven pounds. This wiggling baby kicks, stretches, and pushes. The muscles of the uterus tighten and squeeze. With excitement the mother feels this pushing and pressure. The pushes, called contractions, begin slowly and gradually come closer together. The uterus is now ready to gently and slowly push the baby on his way from his comfortable warm home. The time has come for the baby to be born.

The mother lies on her back. The uterus contracts, then it rests. Then it squeezes again. The baby's head begins to come through the cervix, or the opening of the uterus, and through the vagina to the outside. The shoul-

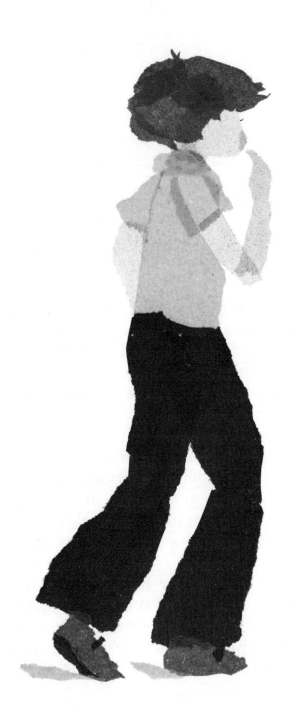

ders and body appear as the baby is born. He takes his first breath and cries. All is well. When the umbilical cord has been clamped and cut, the baby is on his own. A miracle has happened.

Have you ever seen a brand new baby? Usually the skin becomes a very bright pink as soon as the breathing is regular enough to bring in enough oxygen.

Looking at their new baby is very exciting for a mother and father. All sorts of questions come to mind: What was this special little person doing in his pre-earth life such a short time ago? What shall we name him? What will he be like in ten or eleven years? What kind of person will he be as a teenager and as an adult? What kind of parents will we be? And will this precious baby be happy? What problems will he face? And look at those perfect little fingers, and legs, and ears. Oh, what wonderful blessings! What a miracle!

Yes, this is a miracle. Having a baby in the family is exciting. Life will never be the same again for mother or father. Every baby makes a family different. You did. In fact, you probably can't imagine how much you changed the lives of everyone around you. You probably can't fully realize how much you have been loved, as a baby and as you are now.

This is all part of a very long story. You lived for a long time before the day you were born on earth. You learned much in that pre-earth life in the presence of heavenly parents. But there came a time when you needed to come to earth. You needed a body. You needed to live, to learn, and to work—to experience many things, and especially to learn about life and eternity as taught through the gospel of Jesus Christ. It was also important for you to come here to perform gospel ordinances, such as baptism, and later sealing ordinances in the temple for your own family. So this birth of yours was a very important and special event. Every birth is. And when you are a parent and look at a little beautiful baby of your own, you will have seen a miracle come true.

You Are a Very Important Person

Have you ever stopped to think about yourself in comparison with everyone else in the world? How many students are enrolled in your school? How many people do you think live in your community? Do you have any idea how many people live in your country? Now try to imagine how many people live in the world. The number is almost too gigantic to imagine. Yet you are just one person among all these billions of people. Have you ever felt rather insignificant in a big crowd of people, or as you thought about all the people in the world? Have you ever thought that one person "isn't very important?"

Most of us have probably thought we were unimportant at one time or another. Elder Paul

41

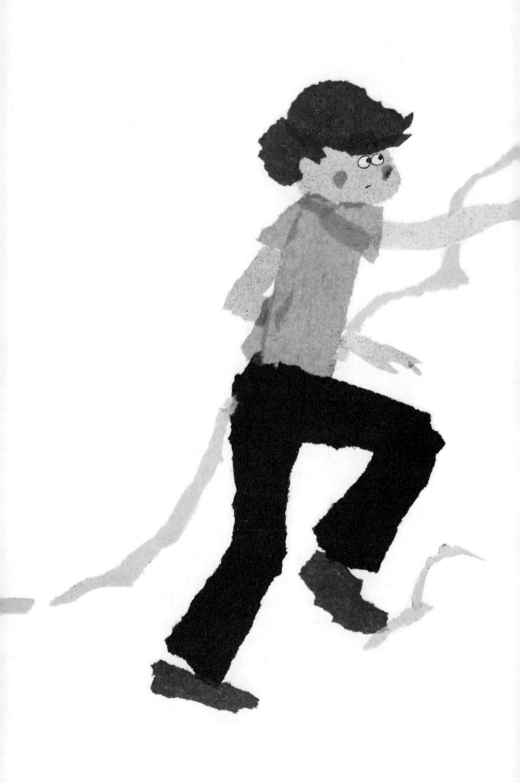

H. Dunn did. One night as he looked up at the stars he thought to himself, "I am one speck on one tiny world that's going around one of the seventy trillion stars. How small and totally insignificant I am." That night, as he unrolled his sleeping bag, a thought came to him with great impact: "I am older than the rocks (for my spirit is eternal). I am more important than all seventy trillion stars (because I am God's son, and they are only his handiwork)." (Paul H. Dunn and Richard M. Eyre, *Goals*, Bookcraft, 1976.)

A son or daughter of God—that's you. You've been given a miraculous body, with the commandment to keep it pure and clean. Give it the care and attention it deserves, and never under any circumstances misuse it or let anyone else abuse it. That body houses the eternal soul of one of God's special children.

If there are times when you don't feel important, stop and remember who you are and how important you are, especially to your Heavenly Father and to your earthly father and mother. Then think about the blessings you have because you were born at this particular time. It didn't just happen by chance. You wanted to come to earth. You wanted a mortal body. You are here for a reason. Knowing these things makes it easier to understand why you belong to your family and someone else belongs to another family.

And so your adventure in life is becoming more exciting every day. Many wonderful things are ahead. You are "writing" the story of your life every day. You yourself make up the script that you will live and act today. This doesn't mean you can have everything you want. You can choose to do many things. You can make some excellent choices or some that are not so good. The choices you make can help you have a happy life and eternity with a worthy companion, or they may result in something less. Never forget that you are a very important person—a child of God.

As you think about life, about yourself, and about what you are doing, think about how important you really are. Don't get too puffed up about it—just think about it to yourself. You deserve the best. This doesn't necessarily mean you will have the best of whatever you think you want right now. But it does mean that you can have the best life. You can have the happiest day—right now, today. You can be happy if you tell yourself you are, and mean it. Be happy because you are alive. Be happy because you know who you are. Be happy because you

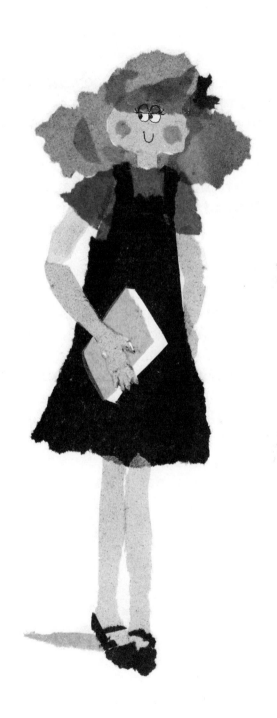

can choose the very best companion for you, to be yours forever.

You can begin right now to look for the best person you can find in all the world to be your forever companion. Settle for no one but the best. But remember also that you have to be the best kind of companion yourself, if you are going to attract that special person. Look carefully and prepare well. Be clean, neat, kind, and good natured, and make yourself grow into the kind of person who can win the love of that very special person you want for an eternal companion. And then you can belong to each other forever by being married to each other in one of the Lord's holy temples, for time and all eternity.

You will because you are you . . . a very special and important person.